So You Had A Stroke

(revised Ed.Jan 2014)

by

Maxwell R Watson

Copyright Max Watson 2011

ISBN: -978-1495489891

Published at Smashwords

And createspace.com

maxwatson@iinet.net.au

I0439489

Dedication

I dedicate this book to my longsuffering wife Christine, you are amazing darling, thank you for sticking with me through all the ups and downs over the past three decades; I love you more than I can ever find words to say.

Disclaimer

I am not attempting to answer every possible question anyone could have, that is simply not possible. Nor am I addressing issues you should not discuss with your own doctor or therapists'. Nor am I some kind of font of all wisdom, because I'm not, I'm just a guy who survived a massive stroke and who wants to encourage other people in that situation to keep going, life is worth living.

Warning

Additionally, I want to encourage all people that are brain injury free to do whatever you need to do to stay that way. If you are an ultra-busy professional, stop, take a life inventory, make whatever changes required ensuring you are healthy, your BMI is under 30, and you are not a walking stroke or heart attack. Eat a healthy balanced diet and if at all possible get some regular exercise.

If you are an Adlerian junky, I urge you to take every safety measure to protect yourself from Brain injury.

Human Brain Facts

1. No pain. There are no pain receptors in the brain, so the brain itself, can feel no pain.
2. Blood vessels. There are 160,000 kilometres of blood vessels in the brain.
3. Fat. The human brain is the fattest organ in the body and may consist of at least 60% fat.
4. Skin. Your skin weighs twice as much as your brain.
5. Water. The brain contains about 75% water.
6. Grey matter. The brain's grey matter is made up of neurons, which gather and transmit signals.
7. Your brain consists of about 100 billion neurons.
8. There are anywhere from 1,000 to 10,000 synapses for each neuron.

Introduction

So, you, or someone close to you, has suffered a stroke! Firstly, I would like to say that I am truly sorry about that. Secondly, I did too; and no, I do not have all the answers for you or anyone. I simply wanted to be able to give people a free resource to help in this difficult time. You probably will have, or soon will have, dozens of questions. I would also highly advise that you contact your local or regional Brain Injury Association for assistance and further information.

I have written this booklet in an attempt to help you understand some of what you have are experiencing. However, the number-one positive thing is that you survived, and you have a life yet to live, enjoy and succeed in.

You may not think that surviving a Stroke is necessarily the best thing in all this, but I assure you that it is, and a whole lot better than the other option. If you are a relative, of a Stroke survivor, you need to understand many things will now possibly change, and I will address some of these issues as I proceed.

I have chosen to ask and answer questions that I had and sadly had to find out for myself.

You will have lots of doctors and therapists telling you many things about yourself that will be very difficult for you to understand and indeed to accept.

You have an injury (called an acquired brain injury or **ABI**) to your brain, and this will mean that things are now different for you or your loved ones.

The level or amount of these differences depends entirely on the area of your brain that has been affected and the amount of damage there is to that affected area.

Doctors will tell you many things, but ultimately, they do not know if you will totally recover or not. The brain is the most complicated organ in the human body, and it has abilities far beyond any current human understanding to make new pathways (that's called neuroplasticity). To read more on neuroplasticity go to.

http://en.wikipedia.org/wiki/Neuroplasticity

It is going to take time for you to understand the full impact of your Stroke. That's OK, no one has the right to tell you things like: "get over it," "just accept the way you are and make the most of your life" and other hurtful and meaningless statements that people sometimes make. We each need to take the time we need to come to terms with surviving a Stroke and what that means to you, and that is different for every single person.

You may well have times of depression because of the effects on your life. I sure did. Just remember **DO NOT** isolate yourself and **DO NOT** make major decisions when in a depressed state. If you realize you are depressed see your doctor **immediately**, **DO NOT** attempt to use other people's prescribed medication, over the counter herbal medicine, illegal drugs or alcohol to "help you get by" or "cope" —They **DO NOT** work and in most cases will only make matters far, far worse.

If you feel like it would be better to have died than survive. Seek help you could well be depressed and in need of help. By the way, those thoughts though appearing real, are, in fact, a lie. Life is good and in time, you will learn how to take full advantage of the time you have to engage in life, family, friends and fun once again.

How will my life change?

This will depend entirely on the extent of any disability you may have following your time in rehabilitation.

You may have to relearn how to do many normal everyday things in order to live an independent life. I had to relearn how to many things myself, even toileting, which is a little embarrassing for a 50-year-old.

You may not be able to go back to your job or business; I highly recommend getting counselling as such a huge change in your life will take some talking and working through. You will need to Hope for the best while planning for the worst, in that you may well believe that you will fully recover – good. Meanwhile, get the necessary equipment to assist you in living. Take your time relearning things that you have done automatically, without thinking, this is a frustrating time, but you can do it.

You may need some retraining before you can go back to any job. Yes, this is very frustrating too, but you need to do what you need to do. E.g. I was only 49 when I suffered a massive stroke and was left with my left side paralysed, we had four teenage children all still living at home with us and all in high school, the Disability Support Pension I was eligible for was just NOT paying the bills. So returning to some kind of paid employment was not really an option, I simply had to find a way to work. (Now and close to 10 years post-stroke and retired, I don't know how I worked that job for five years, but I did.)

You may or may not be able to drive a car again; there are many aids and adaptations that can be installed, both in a car, and in your home, to assist you.

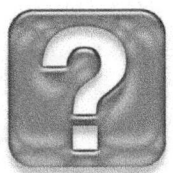

WILL I STILL BE ABLE TO ENJOY SEX?

Yes, there may be some complications. If you are male, you may have some level of impotence, for which you can get help. You may need to be a little creative, but with understanding, love and care; there is no reason that you should not lead a fulfilling sex life.

Relationships and disability (from

http://en.wikipedia.org/wiki/Sexuality_and_disability)

People with disabilities have the same basic human need to form close relationships as do other people. However, Western culture has had a long history of secluding and segregating people with disabilities, greatly inhibiting their ability to meet and socialize with many people. Many people still take it for granted that someone with a disability is either uninterested in romance or sexuality, or is unable to participate in sexual activity.

Stereotypes about disability add to the difficulty and stigma for people with disabilities. Myths about men and women with disabilities have been identified as follows.

- Men and Women with disabilities don't need sex.
- Men and Women with disabilities are not sexually attractive.
- Men and Women with disabilities are 'oversexed.'
- Men and Women with disabilities have more important needs than sex.
- Boys and Girls living with disabilities don't need sexuality education.
- Men and Women who live with disabilities can't have 'real' sex.
- Sex must be spontaneous and/or have a set time.
- Men and Women with disabilities and retardation should not have children and not allowed to have children.

Up to 50% of adults with disabilities are not in any sexual relationship at all, according to one survey.

Dozens of online dating sites specifically aimed at people with disabilities have formed in recent years to fill this void. A 2012 Australian documentary directed by Catherine Scott, _Scarlet Road_, explores another aspect of the void facing people with disabilities, as it shows a sex worker who has specialized for 18 years in a clientele who have disabilities.

DO I BELIEVE EVERYTHING THE DOCTORS AND THERAPISTS TELL ME?

No, They only know what is considered "normal" over a given number of cases. They do not know you, your ability to fight and recover. A personal example:

An Occupational Therapist was trying to convince me to get a special one-handed keyboard for a computer – I steadfastly refused. My reasoning was simple; "I have been using computers for over 25 years; I am fairly good with computers, but I need to be able to sit and use any computer and not be limited to using a "special'" keyboard." As soon as I was released from the rehabilitation hospital. I began the process of re-educating myself in computer usage. I quickly found that having the keyboard at a 45-degree angle to my chair made one-handed typing much easier and created a lot less wrist strain than having the keyboard in a "normal" position. (There are specially designed one-handed keyboards if required. Go to http://www.frogpad.com/ image below)

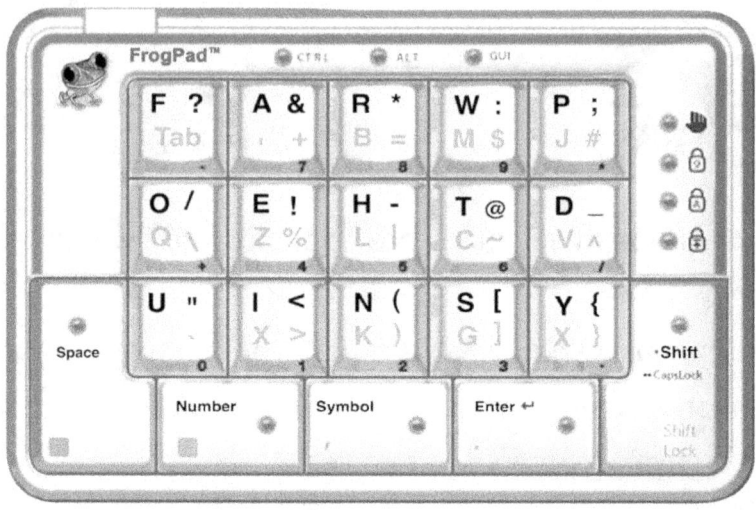

In fact, this booklet was written on a normal Apple MacBook Pro and edited on an average desktop computer using Windows.

WILL I EVER BE "NORMAL" AGAIN?

No-one can answer that question. If indeed, "normal" means anything anyway. You will certainly need to make some life changes, even if your recovery appears to be 100%. You had a stroke – it is not a funny thing that you now live with an ABI. Getting fit, losing weight, etc. are all important aspects of life that you may need to address. Do it? If you have been a workaholic, then that **MUST** be addressed; e.g. I was a workaholic for many, many years. It was a contributing factor to my stroke. Get over it, get help, see a counsellor or a life coach, but stop being a workaholic. If you are reading this and have not had a stroke but can relate to this paragraph, do anything whatsoever to avoid having a stroke; tell your overweight work colleagues to get a handle on their weight. I repeat Do **ANYTHING** NECESSARY TO AVOID A STROKE. If you have never been a person of faith, then explore your spirituality, it is a fact that people with a strong faith live longer and more contented & fulfilled lives than people with no religious faith. If you have no one you feel comfortable in asking about spirituality, contact me and I will put you in touch with someone near you that will help (regardless of where you are in the world); my email address is located on the title page.

I personally believe the most import attitude to embrace is for you to be totally and completely determined to never, never, never give up. I believe this so much I had it tattooed on my arm,

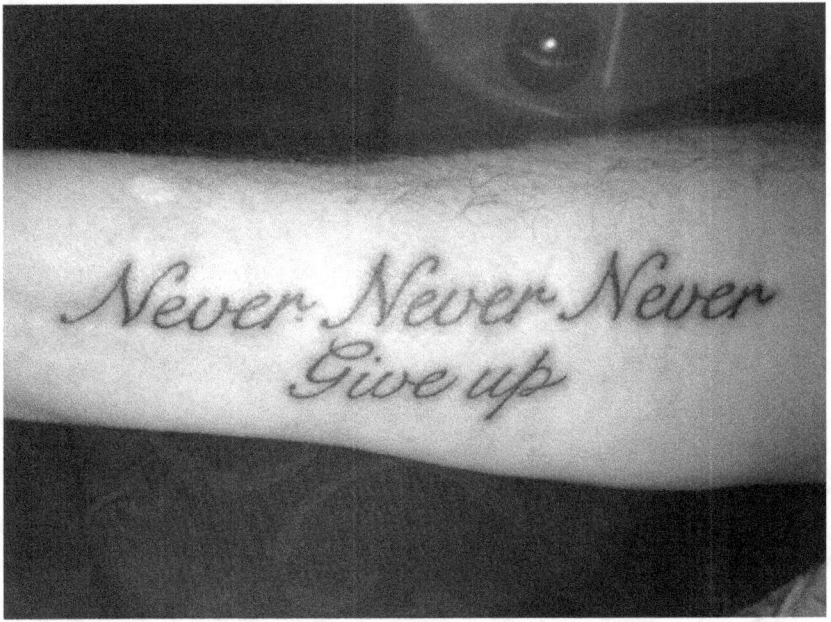

This way, I read my own motto every day: Never, Never, Never Give up!

Understand that you could well experience sea-sawing emotions, even despair of your situation; my emotions were certainly changed due to my stroke. I cry much more easily now, and I sometimes feel embarrassed that a story told in church or a movie makes me cry. Keep focused; life is worth living; you were not meant to die.

If I had not survived my stroke; I would not have seen each of my children graduate high school, would not have witnessed my eldest daughter graduate with her Degree, I would not have walked (I usually say hobbled) two of my girls down the Aisle at their weddings, and I would have never known my Granddaughter Zoe.

Do not think that life is not worth living – because it is so very much worth it. It is vital that you seek out the help you need.

ON DOCTORS/THERAPISTS AND COUNSELLORS

Not every doctor, therapist or counsellor will necessarily be the right one for you. I changed my GP after being at that particular practice for 20 years because I felt he was not doing the best a G.P. could or should do for me. The same goes for Therapists and counsellors. There are varying kinds of counselling and approaches you may find that the first one you see is not necessarily the best option. Do not be afraid to say I want to see someone else. I do know that if you do not address frustration and anger you feel that it will lead to serious problems.

WHAT WILL MY PARTNER DO?

The secret in continuing to live life well is having a dedicated carer/partner, in my case my amazing wife of 33 years, Christine, to say she is amazing is a gross understatement; however, I lack the vocabulary to put into words how amazing she is. She cares for me in every way. She is patient, reassuring and most importantly she encourages me every step of the way. Even as I am about to get an electric wheelchair, my OT thinks it's time, she has that special ability to see the positives and reassures me that it will be OK.

I am a person with a strong faith. I am fully aware that not everyone is; however, I urge you to look at the spiritual side of life. It is a fact that people with a strong faith recover better from traumatic events in life. If you don't know where to begin I suggest you contact you contact the hospital Chaplin. If that is not helpful to you the my emaiol address is on page 1 and I will help.

WHAT HELP IS AVAILABLE TO ME?

There is a huge amount of help available, starting with your local General Practitioner. He or she should be able to handle any medical issues or problems you encounter. Confide in him/her, as this relationship will be vital for you in the future. Therapy on an ongoing basis maybe of benefit to you, or you may get to a point where it is no longer helping you to go forward, and you decide to stop going. Again, this is your decision. Do not stop making decisions for yourself; just be sensible – there may well be times when you need to allow your "significant other" to make decisions for you. An example: I suffered a deep and very dark depression; during that time, I had to allow my wife to make most of the more important decisions.

Another issue is my ABI has meant my hearing has virtually disappeared, to the point that I now have to wear two hearing aids, with which I have a love/hate relationship. I also cannot process complex questions. At some recent medical appointments, I have to allow my wife to do most of the answering of questions, make the decisions, and fill me in later.

Special Note: If you are reading this on behalf of a stroke survivor and their ability to speak has been damaged. Please do not despair, there are ways to learn to communicate again. There are many return to work agencies, I suggest you begin with the one your therapist recommends. In Australia that is usually The Commonwealth Rehabilitation Service... The Brain Injury Association is also extremely helpful and I would very highly recommend you visit www.biansw.org.au and or www.brainfacts.org/ and read everything on that site to help you help yourself or your loved one.

There are numerous disability-focused agencies that can and will help you gain employment. Begin by asking your GP, your local Council should have a list or get a friend to do an Internet search of what is available in your area. Never be backward in coming forward to someone to ask.

A few **MUSTS** in closing: You Must:

- Have a positive attitude
- Choose happiness
- Have your medical needs correctly met. This may mean you have to become the like the squeaky wheel in need of oil.
- Make goals
- Set priorities
- Have sub aims to reach each goal. Step by step; baby steps are quite OK.

- Remember above all else:

Never, Never, Never Give Up

Some resources:

http://drleaf.com/

www.brainfacts.org/

http://www.myhandicap.com

http://www.braininjuryaustralia.org.au/

www.biansw.org.au

http://www.youtube.com/watch?v=SjbX6mDnMwM

http://www.restorative-therapies.com

https://beacon.anu.edu.au

Books to read:

SWITCH ON YOUR BRAIN

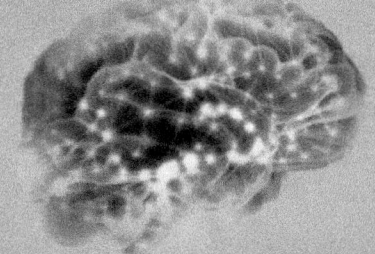

The Key to PEAK HAPPINESS, THINKING, and HEALTH

DR. CAROLINE LEAF

STORIES of PERSONAL TRIUMPH from the FRONTIERS OF BRAIN SCIENCE

The BRAIN that CHANGES ITSELF

Norman Doidge, M.D.

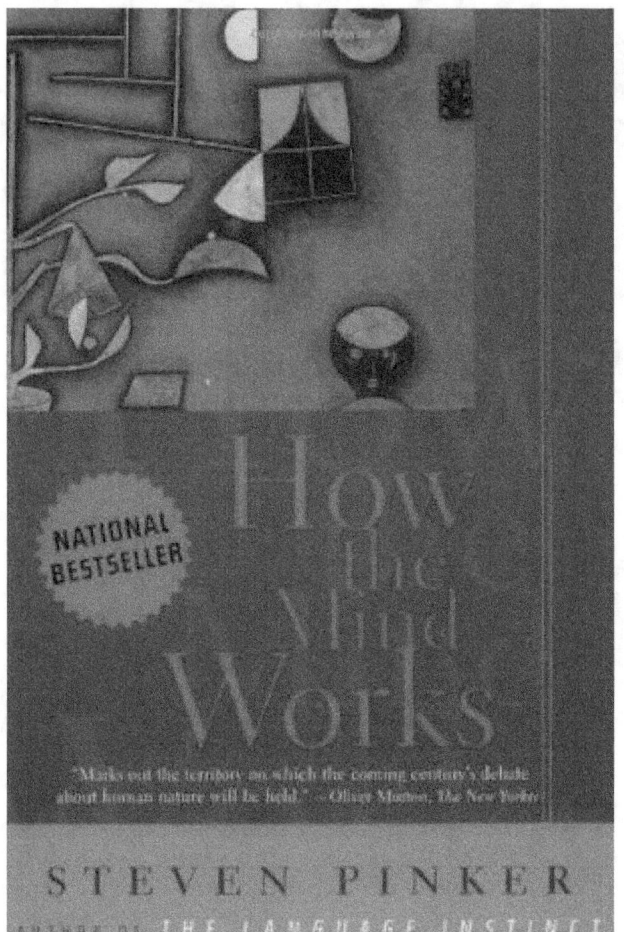

How the Mind Works

"Marks out the territory on which the coming century's debate about human nature will be held." —Oliver Morton, The New Yorker

STEVEN PINKER

AUTHOR OF *THE LANGUAGE INSTINCT*

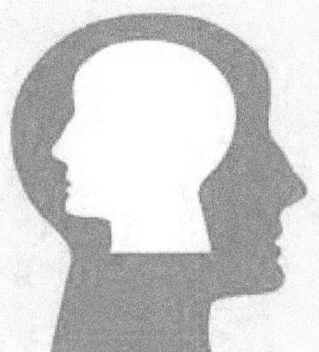

INCOGNITO

THE SECRET LIVES
OF THE BRAIN

DAVID
EAGLEMAN

NATIONAL BESTSELLER